Table of Contents

Chapter 1

Quick action herbs for detoxification

1. Natural Gum Acacia

Produced using the sap of the acacia tree, this substance has been utilized for quite a long time to soothe side effects of the runs by adding mass to solid discharges and enhancing electrolyte ingestion. It is likewise one of a few fixings in Oxy-Powder®. As a hydrocolloid, it is utilized as an emulsifier to balance out and encourage cooperative energy between two fixings which would not ordinarily combine well. [1]

2. Dandelion

For quite a long time, parts of the whole dandelion plant have been utilized to help with an extensive variety of diseases. It advances gut consistency and great hydration levels in the body. What's more, its popular subordinate, dandelion tea, has been utilized to help with joint uneasiness. Dandelion root is utilized as a part of our liver-purging item, Livatrex® in light of the fact that it underpins bile creation, and bile transports toxics out of the body. Dandelion is additionally accepted by some to help the body's invulnerable system. [2]

3. Natural Milk Thistle

This herb has been utilized to help the gallbladder and liver for more than 2,000 years. It has been known not create bile, which thusly enhances digestive capacity. Milk thorn is a dynamic fixing in Livatrex®, which is our most prevalent liver and gallbladder purging item. [3]

4. Dark Walnut

Europeans were initially acquainted with this herb in the 1600's. Three dynamic operators in dark walnut, juglone, tannins, and iodine, make it especially compelling in common wellbeing and health hones. Juglone is the dark walnut's normal resistance component, which battles against unsafe creatures such as microscopic organisms and parasite. Tannins additionally prevent unsafe creatures. Iodine, a fundamental mineral to all life shapes, decreases the lifespan of numerous destructive creatures.

5. Wormwood

The subject of much old stories, wormwood's intense notoriety as a part of absinthe lead to it being banned in the United States for a long time. In spite of the fleeting hiccup, wormwood is back and has been utilized since Egyptian times to battle unsafe living beings, for example, pinworms and roundworms. It has additionally truly been utilized to help with absorption.

6. Cilantro

Cilantro is instrumental in offering the body some assistance with ridding itself of perilous dangerous metals that gather in organ tissues. It is additionally an exceptionally prominent herb that is discussed on practically every cooking appear. Cilantro has characteristic purifying operators that contain mixes which tie to poisonous metals and haul them out of different tissues. [4]

7. Hay Leaf

Botanists have utilized Alfalfa leaf for quite a long time to help with an askindsment of diseases. Numerous trusted that it additionally helped the body battle stomach ulcers furthermore animated a sound hunger.

8. Peppermint

Peppermint has a relieving quality that assists with hacking connected with colds and influenza. It additionally assists with sore throats and sinus bothering. Since it helps likewise helps the body in battling off unsafe life forms, it is a dynamic fixing in lung purifying items like AllerTrex®.

9. Eucalyptus

Eucalyptus is another herb that assists with lung purifying. It has expectorant properties, battles microbes, and assaults infections. It can likewise be utilized as a topical treatment for mid-section blockage and a halted up nose. Native medication profoundly respected it for its quieting, relieving properties.

10. Stinging Nettle

Known for its capacity to oppose microorganisms, it additionally has cancer prevention agent properties. Stinging weed is additionally impervious to systemic redness and swelling and advances ordinary pulse.

Chapter 2

Toxins and Ageing
Maturing, Illness and Repair

Maturing and disease are by and large acknowledged as inescapable as we progress in years, with symptomatic treatment regularly the main accessible choice.

Genuine brokenness is hard to succeed, whether the aftereffect of a traumatic harm, sickness or an inborn issue.

The body is outlined with self-repair components, unless the fragile parity inside of it is upset.

LifeSound gives a powerful and easy to-apply system to empower the body to recalibrate itself and express prior, sound and crucial cell programs. This is accomplished by method for the art of reverberation; reverberation with the hints of wellbeing and essentialness,

Substantial Metals, Chemical Toxins, Disease, Dysfunction and LifeSound

Endless toxics barrage us every day, and our bodies adapt to some of this unsettling influence, however consistent and/or inordinate introduction to toxics might bring about a system over-burden.

Poison over-burden might bring about interruption in our substantial procedures, organs and systems. Genuine sickness or brokenness might create.

LifeSound presents sounds which make a cell smaller scale vibration. This vibration gives the mechanical intends to the physical dislodgement of toxics and pathogens from the body.

Amid the purifying procedure, the body dispenses with the discharged toxics in the typical way (breath, pee, sweat, or defecation).

Particular supplements (or dribbles, if necessary) are prescribed to bolster the body amid the detoxification forms. These are exclusively decided, under the counsel of a medicinal specialist.

LifeSound Supports Optimally Healthy Cellular Programs

Alleviated of toxics, the body is more ready to be adjusted, and indispensable vitality turns out to be more accessible to basic substantial procedures, as opposed to being "squandered" during the time spent determining toxics. The normal result of this is the self-recuperating components of the body are re-built up.

Cell wellbeing, alongside DNA wellbeing, develops as an all the more fundamentally solid body.

LifeSound-related wellbeing upgrades are seen as enhanced memory, better rest designs, enhanced assimilation, adjusted safe system, illness, agony and infirmity determination, capacity change, and that's just the beginning.

Chapter 3

The role of detoxification

We tend to manhandle our body in the ordinary course of life. We subject it to undesirable garbage nourishment and beverages that put a great deal of weight on the inside organs. On top of it, inactive way of life combined with absence of activity and a boisterous every day life makes physiological pandemonium showed as physical and mental issues.

It is crucial that we give our body some reprieve and abundantly required rest, which is the place the significance of detox falsehoods. The detoxification process works by moving the center from metabolizing undesirable sustenances towards cell recovery and inner purifying of the body.

The significance of detox routine is that it serves to advance the admission of nourishments and beverages that are either helpful in flushing out toxics or are the building squares of the body cells. In this way, rather than straining to breakdown intemperate sugars, fats and contaminations the body shifts into a resting mode by totally evading such sustenances and beverages. Cancer prevention agents, which have been observed to be the way to assurance from unsafe free radicals unreservedly flowing in the body, are particularly joined in detox diets.

While our eating regimen is in our grasp what is not is contamination. Aside from natural contamination we additionally ingest toxics through pesticide loaded foodstuffs and beverages bound with to a great degree unsafe metallic mixes. While we can't do much about natural contamination, we can endeavor to expend naturally delivered and other invigorating foodstuffs. In any case, even this is insufficient to recuperate the body adequately. The significance of detox lies in the way that it can get rid of the toxics aggregated inside of the body that is past the span of typical purging procedures.

Detox eating regimens might invoke pictures of dull and bland weight control plans or amazing starvation. Be that as it may, you require not fall back on any of these. The reality of the matter is that there are sure detox consumes less calories that have a tendency to be exceptionally prohibitive like, getting by on fluid eating routine for some time et cetera. Be that as it may, a fundamental comprehension of the significance of detox would uncover that evacuation of each one of those sustenances and different segments that stretch the body is its essential point. Thus, by only after an essential and straightforward eating routine arrangement you can offer your body some assistance with cleansing itself so it is restored to its previous wellbeing.

There are water diets, lemon detox eating regimens and some more. These are somewhat extreme on the body and may not be some tea. Thus, for wellbeing in some tea, settle on detox tea. The significance of detox tea can't be thought little of as it is greatly important as a guide to the kidneys and the liver, which are the essential organs dealing with the discharge process.

It is vital that we comprehend the significance of detox and utilize it to free the tissues of the contaminations that we have a tendency to collect after some time so that the body might be reinvigorated and restored and prepared to confront new difficulties.

Chapter 4

Importance of detoxification

Are detox programs better than average for you? There is by all accounts an equivalent measure of notices and suggestions for detoxing, which can make it mistaking for the eventual detox health food nut. While it is conceivable to fail to understand the situation, the length of you take care of business you'll be helping yourself in a few unique ways. We've laid out a portion of the advantages you can expect by taking after a portion of the all the more very much kindsed out detox programs out there.

detox helps vitality

1. Helps Your Energy

Numerous detox program adherents report feeling more enthusiastic. This would bode well on the grounds that while you're detoxing you're halting the flood of the things that made you require a detox in any case. By removing the sugar, caffeine, trans fat, immersed fat, and supplanting them with new foods grown from the ground, you'll be getting a characteristic jolt of energy, one that comes without a resultant accident. It's key to stay very much hydrated while on any detox program, and that can likewise be a wellspring of expanded vitality on the off chance that you commonly don't get enough water for the duration of the day.

2. Frees the Body of Any Excess Waste

The greatest thing that detoxing assists with is permitting the body to free itself of any overabundance waste it's been putting away. Most detox projects are intended to invigorate the body to cleanse itself, offering the liver some assistance with doing its thing and additionally the kidneys and colon. Purging the colon is an imperative part of the detoxing process since those toxics need to leave the body, and a went down colon can make them be reintroduced into the body, as opposed to leaving as arranged. Staying with leafy foods even after the detox system is finished is a decent approach to keep things moving.

3. Assists with Weight Loss

It's anything but difficult to perceive how a detox eating regimen would make you shed pounds in the short term, yet a more advantageous approach to take a gander at it would be to build up long haul dietary patterns, and free yourself of horrible propensities. Ordinarily it is the extraordinary decrease in calories and fast weight reduction that is centered around, particularly in the media. In any case, these transient results won't last in the event that you don't make it a point to supplant awful sustenances with great, and utilize your recently discovered vitality to practice increasingly and be more dynamic by and large.

4. More grounded Immune System

When you detox the body you free up your organs to work the way they ought to. This gives your invulnerable system a help since you'll have the capacity to assimilate supplements better, including Vitamin C. A large number of the herbs you take while on a detox will help the lymphatic system, which assumes a major part in keeping you solid and terminating on all chambers. Numerous detox programs additionally concentrate on light activities which course lymph liquid through the body and helps it to deplete, fortifying your insusceptible system all the while.

skin advantages of detoxing

5. Enhanced Skin

Your skin is your biggest organ, so it just bodes well that it would demonstrate positive results from a detox program. One approach to offer your detoxing endeavors some assistance with being to take a sauna to help the body sweat out extra toxics. You can expect clearer, smoother skin toward the end of your detox arrangement. It's additionally been accounted for that detoxing can help with skin inflammation, in spite of the fact that the condition might exacerbate before it improves as the toxics are discharged. You might find that your skin tingles or gets inconsistent before clearing up, however this is a piece of the procedure and is an indication that you're in good shape with your project.

6. Better Breath

Take after a detox program that incorporates a colon rinse since those toxics should be discharged from the body. It's been conjectured that one benefactor to terrible breath is a went down colon. When you can get it out and get your digestive system working great once more, you might find that your breath makes strides. Know that your breath might really decline amid the detoxing process, however when it's done it will be better. This is characteristic, and happens as toxics are discharged from the body.

7. Advances Healthy Changes

It's difficult to change a long-standing propensity, and a detox program – regardless of to what extent – is one approach to put a wedge between your old ways and your new ones. On the off chance that you have addictions to sugar, caffeine, singed, or crunchy nourishments you can utilize a detox system to help you slaughter those longings. Frequently in the event that you simply attempt to stop eating those nourishments or drinking those refreshments you'll have constrained achievement, and do a reversal to your old ways. Be that as it may, on the off chance that you purge the body and supplant those nourishments with more beneficial decisions, you can retrain yourself and will probably adhere to your new propensities.

8. Clearer Thinking

A decent detox project will give careful consideration to your perspective amid the wash down. The utilization of reflection is frequently prescribed as an approach to get back in contact with your body amid this season of cleansing and purging of toxics. Detox devotees regularly say that they lose that feeling of fogginess, and can think more unmistakably amid a detox than when not on it. It bodes well, since a large portion of the sugar-filled and fat-filled sustenances that encompass us every day will make us feel dormant and can calculate vigorously the nature of our reasoning.

9. Better Hair

When you can see your hair, it's as of now viewed as dead, as the greater part of its development happens inside of the hair follicle. This is the reason it's vital to keep your body working at its maximum capacity through a normal detoxing methodology. At the point when your hair can become uninhibited by inner toxics you'll see and feel the distinction in your hair. In numerous cases hair gets shinier, and feels milder to the touch. Detoxing isn't sufficient to stop male example sparseness, yet numerous report that their hair develops all the more rapidly, an indication of more advantageous hair.

10. Lighter Feeling

One of the reported advantages of detoxing is a sentiment being lighter. There are a few reasons why this would be the situation, particularly in the event that you'll be doing a colon wash down as a major aspect of the system. When you quit eating sustenances that measure you down, and supplant them with new natural leafy foods, a lighter feeling will undoubtedly happen. It's likewise critical not to gorge while detoxing, which will yield a lighter feeling too, and will give you the vitality you've been absent.

11. Anti Aging Benefits

The consistent blast of toxics that the body needs to manage is one contributing component to the maturing process. By lessening the measure of free radical harm done to the body, you're going to see fleeting advantages, as well as long haul advantages in an expanded life span. When you complete your detox program, it's critical not to go right back to the way of life that was creating the poisonous quality. Adhering to an enhanced eating routine and getting day by day action are incredible approaches to ensure that you feel great every snippet of your life.

12. Enhanced Sense of Wellbeing

When you detox, you feel great, and when you feel great, great things happen. Detoxing is regularly utilized deliberately to get in shape or to begin another eating routine arrangement, yet truly there's no preferable reason over just to feel better. When you set the stage for wellbeing, you are going to enhance all parts of your life, and you ought to see better connections, better efficiency at work, and a newly discovered or reestablished way of life.

Chapter 5

Traditional ways to detox

For a large number of years the Chinese have honed various detoxification techniques intended to oust toxics and take equalization back to the body. On the off chance that you are keen on detoxifying your body, consider drinking Chinese detox tea, going in for measuring or meridian decrease treatment, or wearing detox foot cushions.

Chinese Detox Tea

The Chinese use herbs to clean the liver, kidneys, lungs and blood. Drinking detox tea frequently will help you feel more settled and give you expanded vitality and clearer skin. The teas contain various strong herbs, for example, red clover, honeysuckle blossom, dandelion root and ginger root. Joined, these herbs advance the flushing of toxics consumed by your body through the earth, smoke, liquor, caffeine and that's only the tip of the iceberg.

Measuring

Measuring, a by and large effortless detox method the Chinese have drilled for centuries, has spread to whatever remains of the world as of late. Like needle therapy, measuring fortifies blood course and treats colds, diseases and muscle and joint torment. The expert will put mugs made out of solid glass specifically on your skin to make suction. Pumps will expand the suction, and your skin inside the container will rise. The suction and weight free up blockages and let your vitality stream.

Scratching

Meridian Tapper

Chinese holds that the body contains several meridians, or vitality focuses. The meridian tapper process clears your meridian ways and expels waste from somewhere down in your muscles. The expert uses an uncommon meridian tapper to clear the way, and raised wounds will show up where your blood had beforehand stagnated. On the off chance that your body is in equalization, the tapper won't create purple welts.

Your body has 360 needle therapy focuses - a considerable lot of which are found in the soles of the feet - where toxics can get away. Chinese foot reflexology keeps up that these focuses associate with comparing parts in rest of the body. Place Chinese foot detox mortars on your feet overnight; the cushions draw the toxics out through the needle therapy focuses while you rest. The cushions will seem darker in the morning, intelligent of the toxics they have drawn out. With expanded utilize, the cushions ought to indicate dynamically lighter recoloring.

Scratching is another Chinese detox process went for enhancing dissemination and vitality stream in your body. Before starting the treatment, touch your skin with oil. The expert will rub the parts of your body requiring incitement to enhance what upsets you. Normally scratched territories incorporate the back, mid-section, arms, shoulder bones and legs. Small red or purple spots that look like rashes will show up on the scratched territory. In spite of the appearance despite what might be expected, the procedure is additionally moderately effortless; the spots show stagnate blood loaded with toxics. After the method, you ought to feel better blood dissemination and in addition alleviation from cerebral pains and sinus torment, among others.

Chapter 6

The process of detoxification

Getting a handle on slow or of sync? Battling with skin issues, a throbbing painfulness, or digestive issues? Can't get in shape? It may be the ideal opportunity for a body detox.

Honed for quite a long time by societies around the globe — including ayurvedic and Chinese solution systems — detoxification is about resting, cleaning and supporting the body from the back to front. By uprooting and killing toxics, then nourishing your body with solid supplements, detoxifying can shield you from sickness and reestablish your capacity to keep up ideal wellbeing.

How does detoxification work?

Essentially, detoxification implies cleaning the blood. This is finished by expelling polluting influences from the blood in the liver, where toxics are prepared for disposal. The body additionally wipes out toxics through the kidneys, digestion systems, lungs, lymph and skin. Be that as it may, when this system is bargained, polluting influences aren't appropriately separated and each cell in the body is unfavorably influenced.

A detox system can help the body's regular purging procedure by:

1. Resting the organs through fasting;

2. Empowering the liver to drive toxics from the body;

3. Advancing disposal through the entrails, kidneys and skin;

4. Enhancing flow of the blood; and

5. Refueling the body with sound supplements.

"Detoxification works since it addresses the requirements of individual cells, the littlest units of human life," says Peter Bennett, N.D., co-creator of 7-Day Detox Miracle with Stephen Barrie, N.D., and Sara Faye.

How would you know whether you have to detoxify?

Bennett recommends that everybody ought to detox at any rate once per year. In any case, Bennett alerts against detoxing for nursing moms, kids, and patients with incessant degenerative sicknesses, tumor or tuberculosis. Counsel your social insurance specialist on the off chance that you have questions about whether detoxing is a good fit for you.

Today, with more toxics in the earth than any time in recent memory, "it's basic to detox," says Linda Page, N.D., Ph.D., the creator of Detoxification. Page suggests detoxing for side effects, for example,

Signs which show detox is working

Unexplained weariness

Drowsy disposal

Bothered skin

Hypersensitivities

Second rate contaminations

Puffy eye or sacks under the eyes

Bloating

Menstrual issues

Mental disarray

How would you begin a detox?

In the first place, alleviate up your poison burden. Take out liquor, espresso, cigarettes, refined sugars and soaked fats, all of which go about as toxics in the body and are deterrents to your recuperating process. Additionally, minimize utilization of concoction based family unit cleaners and individual social insurance items (chemicals, shampoos, antiperspirants and toothpastes), and substitute regular choices.

Another hindrance to great wellbeing is anxiety, which triggers your body to discharge stress hormones into your system. While these hormones can give the "adrenaline surge" to win a race or meet a due date, in substantial sums they make toxics and back off detoxification catalysts in the liver. Yoga, Qigong and contemplation are straightforward and resetting so as to compel approaches to alleviate stress your physical and mental responses to the inescapable anxiety life will bring.

Which detox project is ideal for you?

There are numerous detoxification projects and detox formulas, contingent upon your individual needs. Numerous projects take after a 7-day plan in light of the fact that, as Bennett clarifies, "it takes the body time to clean the blood." His project includes fasting on fluids for two days, trailed by a painstakingly arranged five-day detox eating routine to permit the digestive system to rest. Page prescribes a 3-7 day squeeze quick (drinking just crisp leafy foods squeezes and water) as a powerful approach to discharge toxics.

Here are our five most loved detox diets:

1. Basic Fruit and Veggie Detox

2. Smoothie rinse

3. Juice Cleanse

4. Sugar Detox

5. Hypoallergenic Detox

Main 10 approaches to offer your body some assistance with detoxifying

After a detoxification program, you can purge your body every day with these eating routine, supplements and way of life practices:

1. **Eat a lot of fiber,** including cocoa rice and naturally developed new products of the soil. Beets, radishes, artichokes, cabbage, broccoli, spirulina, chlorella, and kelp are fantastic detoxifying sustenances.

2. **Wash down and secure the liver by taking herbs,** for example, dandelion root, burdock and milk thorn, and drinking green tea.

3. **Take vitamin C,** which helps the body produce glutathione, a liver exacerbate that heads out toxics.

4. **Drink no less than two quarts of water a day.**

5. **Inhale profoundly to permit oxygen to course all the more totally through your system.**

6. **Change stress by underscoring positive feelings.**

7. **Rehearse hydrotherapy by cleaning up for five minutes,** permitting the water to keep running on your back. Take after with cool water for 30 seconds. Do this three times, and after that get into bed for 30 minutes.

8. **Sweat in a sauna** so your body can dispense with squanders through sweat.

9. **Dry-brush your skin** or attempt detox foot spas/foot showers to evacuate toxics through your pores. Uncommon brushes are accessible at common items stores.

10. What is the most imperative approach to detoxify? "Exercise," says Bennett. "Yoga or hop restricting are great. One hour consistently." Also attempt Qigong, a hand to hand fighting based activity system that incorporates practices particularly to detoxify or purging, and in addition numerous different activities with particular medical advantages.

Chapter 7

Physical and mental efficiency with detoxification

"Everybody has a doctor inside him or her; we simply need to help it in its work. The common recuperating power inside of every one of us is the best drive in getting great. Our nourishment ought to be our pharmaceutical. Our drug ought to be our nourishment. Be that as it may, to eat when you are wiped out is to sustain your ailment."

At the point when a creature, for example, a puppy or feline, is wiped out, its regular impulse is to decline sustenance. At the point when the emergency is over, and the inner mending work has been expert, the voracity will return actually, voluntarily.

The human creature likewise has a fasting nature, much the same as that of different creatures. Developmental adjustment has made our bodies extremely effective at putting away vitality holds, and drawing upon them when nourishment supplies are rare.

Fasting is as old as humankind, maybe even more established. As far back as should be obvious, men have been fasting for some reason. It is by all accounts an all inclusive practice.

The antiquated Greeks were awesome professors in fasting. Hippocrates advacated it, as is appeared in the above citation. Plato said that he fasted for more prominent physical and mental effectiveness. Aristotle, his understudy, additionally fasted. Both Galen and Avicenna additionally recommended fasts for their patients.

Purposes and Benefits of Fasting

Essentially, there are two kinds of purposes or targets for fasting. Men quick for either otherworldly or physical reasons, and both are just as legitimate.

Profoundly, fasting offers us some assistance with transcending our dependence and connection to sustenance, and to understand that man doesn't live by bread alone. The brain gets clearer, and otherworldly mindfulness extends. Liberated from satisfying physical appetite, one can then turn one's regard for encouraging the psyche and soul. Otherworldly experts like Pythagoras wouldn't concede any supporter into their higher teachings unless they had initially sanitized themselves through fasting.

Physically, fasting empowers the living being to detoxify and clean house. Since by far most of illnesses are created via autointoxication, fasting has colossal helpful advantages. It additionally gives the digestive organs a highly required rest.

For all fevers and maladies in the intense emergency stage, Hippocrates recommended either a strict quick with only water or therapeutic teas, or an extremely slim fluid eating routine. Fasting is additionally prescribed for colds and influenza, joint pain and stiffness, digestive protests, and all humoral and metabolic issue.

Investigative analyses led on research facility mice have demonstrated that serious confinement of caloric admission significantly develops their lifespan. Since this is fundamentally what fasting will be, fasting holds awesome guarantee forever expansion.

The Physiology of Fasting

For whatever length of time that we're alive, the Innate Heat, or metabolic flame, is constantly dynamic. What's more, the length of this metabolic flame is blazing, it must expend something for fuel.

Typically, this Innate Heat or metabolic flame is sustained by supplements from the sustenance we eat. Yet, when we quick, we remove this external supply of fuel, and the metabolic flame starts to feast upon the body's own particular inward saves. The body's own particular Inner Physician is stirred, and the human living being, in its unbounded mending astuteness, begins to tidy house and consume the dross.

What is minimum key to the life and strength of the creature is devoured initially, for example, toxics, squanders, and unnecessary grim humors. The Inner Physician knows definitely where to go, what to metabolize and dispense with, and how to dispose of it. This is the procedure of autolysis. In this sense, fasting has been portrayed as an operation without surgery.

Fasting gives your digestive organs a quite required rest. Rather than processing nourishment, their digestive emissions and proteins can serve to process, kill and take out dangerous squanders from the body through the GI tract. Boss among these discharges is bile, which is emitted by the liver and nerve bladder.

Contingent upon where the toxics and dismal humors have been held in the body, they will begin to create different signs and manifestations as this waste is disposed of and went off:

Head/Brain: cerebral pains, discombobulation, vertigo, wooziness, unsteadiness.

Nose, Sinuses: wheezing, runny nose, tingling, stinging, post nasal dribble.

Throat: soreness or choking, raspiness, scratchiness

Lungs: mid-section blockage, wheezing, mucus releases, foul breath smells

Skin: rashes, skin break out, pustules; over the top or anomalous sweating; odd stenches

Stomach: acrid or anxious stomach, stomach cramping, burping, awful breath

Liver: sore eyes, intense taste in mouth, pallid composition, torment or distension under

the ribs on the right side.

Nerve Bladder: colic, fit, delicacy or agony underneath the liver range.

Digestion tracts: putrid gas, cramping, loose bowels, spastic colon or touchy entrail.

Kidneys: low back agony and shortcoming, weakness; regular pee, frequently dire;

firmly hued or noticing pee.

For the most part, the all the more as of late obtained toxics and collections of grim matter will be the first to be gone off, trailed by more established and all the more long-standing ones, backtracking backward request of procurement. Likewise, the day's detoxification tends to begin in the morning with head manifestations, and by and large works its way down the body.

The purifying and detoxification manifestations, and the loss of weight and bulk, are the most serious and extraordinary for the initial three days. Inside of these initial three days, vitality levels additionally have a tendency to be least and generally hazardous. After this starting three day period, a change happens in the body's inner vitality economy, called ketosis, in which the living being changes over to the more effective blazing of its fat stores to fulfill its essential vitality needs. At that point, the vitality levels improve.

Amid a quick, the living being detoxifies itself amid the night, leaving a thick, foul, intense tasting deposit on the tongue in the morning. After emerging, it's ready to the restroom with a spoon or tongue scrubber and scratch this buildup off. Precautionary measures for Fasting

Before leaving on a quick, it's great to talk it over with somebody who's fasted some time recently, listening to their story, so you have a superior thought of what's in store. A short quick of three days or less is a genuinely straightforward issue, and can be attempted without an excess of consideration or concern.

In any case, long fasts, for more than three days, are an alternate matter. For these, it's a smart thought to check with your doctor to survey regardless of whether you're ready to proceed with it physically, particularly in the event that you have wellbeing conditions like asthma or kinds 2 diabetes that have traded off your fundamental wellbeing or digestion system. It's additionally a smart thought to have your fasting program composed and observed by a comprehensive medicinal services proficient.

One thing that is basic while fasting is to drink a lot of liquids. These incorporate water, home grown teas and, on account of juice fasting, leafy foods/vegetable juices. Thus the Expulsive Virtue of the Water component is utilized to help the purging and detoxification process.

Back in Hippocrates' day, the majority of the fasting that was done was water fasting, in which noithing however water was devoured. This is the easiest type of fasting, as well as the most serious, in light of the fact that it makes stringent requests on the life form to process and metabolize superfluities and draw all alone inner vitality holds.

These days, water fasting might be okay for short fasts of three days or less, yet it's by and large not educated for fasts with respect to longer length of time. Different misuse pervasive in the present day world, for example, ecological contamination; refined, devitalized, supplement drained sustenances; garbage nourishments and gorging; and medication and substance misuse have made advanced man constitutioanlly weaker and less impervious to the rigors of exceptional detoxification.

Before choosing to attempt a long quick, one ought to get a spotless bill of fundamental wellbeing from a doctor or all encompassing social insurance proficient. The inquiry is: After drawn out fasting has evacuated all that is lethal, dreary and pointless, will regardless you have the fundamental protected quality and resistance left to maintain yourself through the recovery and recuperation process? Numerous whose general wellbeing condition is excessively fragile or once-over would be better ready to handle an augmented quick on the off chance that they first went on a project of tonification and established change in advance.

Kinds of Fasts and Cleansing Diets

Fasts and purging eating regimens are of various kinds. They are attempted for a wide range of purposes and destinations.

A basic quick doesn't surpass over a day or two long, and is attempted when one feels heartburn, absence of hunger, being under the climate, or unwell. In its least complex structure, it comprises only of avoiding a feast, typically supper. Notwithstanding water, herb teas might be smashed that are particular to the condition you're attempting to succeed; with processing of nourishment no more essential, the living being is allowed to get up to speed with back recuperating work. Hippocrates endorsed straightforward fasts in all fevers and intense illnesses in the emergency stage.

Juice fasting is the standard present day technique for taking care of fasts of longer length of time, where a more profound and more exhaustive purging and detoxification is sought. Leafy foods juices, regularly weakened 50/50 with immaculate water, alkalinize the system and velocity up detoxification while giving a base level of calories and supplements to manage vitality; then again, ketosis, or the body's delving into its own fat and vitality stores, isn't as exceptional. Likewise, foods grown from the ground juices, legitimately picked, can be helpful in numerous constant and degenerative conditions, and help the recuperating process. In the initial a few days of a juice quick, the entrails are scrubbed with douches or colonics; this incredibly diminishes the harmful burden on the body, and keeps toxics from old fecal squanders held in the colon from being reabsorbed into the body and the circulation system.

Purifying eating regimens include eating daintily of nourishment that is extremely immaculate, basic, adjusted and simple to process. This accommodates the body's essential vitality and wholesome needs while permitting purging and detoxification to happen. Purifying weight control plans are extremely valuable for those whose constitutions are excessively sensitive or once-over, making it impossible to withstand the speedier, more radical detoxification of a water or squeeze quick.

Numerous purifying weight control plans use different kinds of gruels or porridges. In Ayurvedic medication, a gruel of mung beans or lentils with rice, called kitcharee, is utilized. Chinese prescription uses a rice gruel called congee. In Greek Medicine, the customary planning is ptisan, a kinds of grain water or gruel.

By modifying the proportion of grain to water, or by either straining the grain water or leaving the grain grains in the ptisan, it can be acclimated to practically any wanted consistency. The immense estimation of grain is that it's supporting, simple to process, and calming and emollient to the GI tract, with no lingering astringency that may disturb colic or bloating.

In intense emergencies and fevers, just the fluid, strained ptisan is utilized. For normal detoxification purposes, a soupy gruel is utilized. In the event that a more extensive nourishing base is wanted, root or verdant vegetables, ocean vegetables, herbs, or beans and heartbeats can likewise be cooked into the ptisan; this additionally makes for a decent move back to a common eating regimen.

Upgrading the Cleansing and Detoxification

While fasting, there are various helpful measures that can be taken to upgrade the purifying and detoxification process. The most famous and basic ones are as per the following:

Anointing, oleation, oil rub: Massaging the entire body with fragrant sedated oils enhances the course and detoxification of blood and lymph and upgrades the dumping of waste matter into the GI tract for disposal.

Castor oil: An awesome detoxifier; draws out discharge and toxics. Drink one to two tablespoons, flushed down with lemon water, to scrub the entrails around evening time before resigning, or back rub generously into the stomach area and pelvis to release up and detoxify the guts. Knead into the liver or nerve bladder ranges to straightforwardness sanitization emergencies in these organs.

Dirt: Clay is a mineral whose negative ionic accuse chelates of and draws out emphatically charged acidic toxics. Before utilizing, mud needs some time, preferrably several hours, in a watery situation to ionize legitimately. Blend anyplace from a couple squeezes to a quarter teaspoon of dry powdered mud into some water and let stand for two or three hours before drinking. Mud glue can be put on rashes, abcesses, bubbles and other skin emissions to draw out toxics and rush their determination.

Herb teas: An askindsment of various herb teas can be taken to help the living being in the cleaning and detoxification work it's attempting to finish amid fasting. Subsequent to the body is as of now in a purifying mode, firmly eliminative or laxative herbs aren't required; tender detoxifiers work best.

Purifications and colonics: Cleansing the colon is a smart thought, particularly for a more drawn out quick, since it keeps toxics from old held fecal matter from being reabsorbed into the body and the circulatory system. On the off chance that this is your first quick, or your first colon scrub, it's a smart thought to have it professionally done by an all encompassing medicinal services proficient, as the detoxification responses can be emotional. A progression of a few bowel purges to rinse the colon toward the start of a broadened quick is exceptionally useful. For more data about colon purging, see Hygienic Purification Therapies in the Therapies segment.

Other hygienic refinement treatments, similar to emesis, or remedial heaving, or diaphoresis, or sweating, are likewise extremely accommodating in conjunction with fasting and sanitization administrations where demonstrated. These are best done under the direction and supervision of an all encompassing human services proficient who's gifted and experienced in such work, to appropriately survey the dangers, signs and potential advantages.

Breaking a Fast

The most fundamentally vital part of a quick is the manner by which you end it, or break it. Any blockhead can quick, yet breaking it legitimately is a craftsmanship, and not all that simple. The body must make a steady, orderly move back to a typical eating routine. On the off chance that a drawn out quick isn't broken legitimately, toxics and fecal matter can recongest the gut, and the circulatory system, and every one of the advantages of the quick are invalidated.

For breaking a quick, ptisan is exceptionally helpful. On the principal day after a drawn out juice quick, drink just the strained grain water. On the second day, a slender, soupy gruel is best, and on the third day, a thicker gruel can be had. On the fourth day, you can cook in lentils and vegetables too, and on the fifth day, you can about-face to your typical eating routine.

On the off chance that you can save an ideal opportunity to do as such, invest as much energy trasitioning back to your typical eating regimen as you did fasting. Keep in mind: The wheels of Nature granulate gradually, however extremely well. On the off chance that your solid discharges don't return immediately, simply hold up a couple of days; it sets aside time for them to be restored. Cholerics might need to temper their fretfulness with regards to breaking a quick in the event that they're not going to invalidate every one of the advantages picked up.

The Optimum Timing of Fasting

The primary tenet in timing a quick is that of need, and of listening to your body. A quick is demonstrated at whatever point danger in the body is heading towards an emergency. In the event that side effects like an icy, poor ravenousness, or acid reflux show up, a short, therapeutic quick is demonstrated.

At the point when arranging a more broad or delayed quick, one ought to pay regard to the season of the year and the period of the Moon. A delayed quick ought to be embraced in a season in which the climate is neither excessively hot nor excessively frosty: in the spring, after the last chilly spells of winter have finished; or in the early fall, before the principal cool fronts of drawing closer winter.

Chapter 8

Best detox diets

The association between the body and the psyche is a manifestly obvious one, with the way your body feels having huge influence in how your mind capacities and regardless of whether you encounter a condition of prosperity. Keeping it free of toxics, free radicals, and other frightful things that can wind up in our inner parts is basically to keeping up a sound life. You'll see that with a significant number of these detox nourishments the street to refinement experiences the liver, and inspiring it to full limit can have a few enduring advantages all through the body.

Artichokes

Artichokes offer the liver capacity taking care of business, which thusly some assistance with willing help your body cleanse itself of toxics and different things it doesn't have to survive. It ups the liver's creation of bile, and since bile separates sustenances which helps your body utilize the supplements inside them, an expansion in bile generation is commonly something to be thankful for.

Beside the greater part of the advantages to your liver, it's additionally loaded with fiber, protein, magnesium, folate, and potassium. It's essentially a decent nourishment to add to your eating regimen to stay normal, stay solid, and keep your liver joyfully doing its occupation.

asparagus

Asparagus

In spite of being a delectable veggie asparagus positions very on the detox-o-meter. Not just does it detoxify the body, it can offer you wage the counter maturing fight, some assistance with protecting you from getting malignancy, help your heart to stay solid, and is a general calming nourishment.

It's likewise known not with liver seepage, which may seem like an awful thing, yet since the liver is in charge of sifting through the poisonous materials in the nourishment and beverages we devour, anything that moves down its waste is not helping you.

Avocados

Due to its fiber and cancer prevention agent tally this is a nourishment that is making it onto more detox records. At first numerous shied far from them in light of they're high in fat, yet following the time when the distinction between great fats and terrible fats turn out to be all the more regularly known, they are currently getting the admiration they merit.

Try not to believe that the guacamole you can add to your dinner at a fast food eatery for 50 pennies more is going to do the detox trap. Decide on natural avocados and expend them with no different fixings to get the full advantage of their sound substance.

beets

Beets

You might just see beets when you arrange a Greek serving of mixed greens, however you ought to attempt to incorporate them into your consistent menu, and unquestionably lift some up in case you're going on a detox diet. There are such a large number of various advantages to them, it's anything but difficult to see why they are frequently specified as a super nourishment.

When you're making so as to detox they will help beyond any doubt that the toxics you're getting out really make it out of your body. Numerous detox scrubs turn out badly when toxics are reintroduced to the body since they don't make it such a distance out. Beets additionally help with free-radicals, making them an against tumor help.

broccoli

Broccoli

You're most likely tired of seeing broccoli appear everywhere at whatever point wellbeing nourishment is specified. In any case, that is simply because it packs a dietary punch in a little tree molded vegetable. Why does it have a place on your detox sustenance shopping list? It particularly works with the compounds in your liver to transform toxics into something your body can take out effectively.

In case you're stuck for courses on the most proficient method to improve broccoli taste take a stab at switching up the way you cook it, or consider eating it crude. Be that as it may, don't microwave it or it won't have the same detox properties.

cabbage

Cabbage

Try not to let the trend Cabbage Soup Detox Diet throw you off base with this accommodating vegetable. Like most things that circulate around the web this eating regimen has some truth to it, yet you don't need to go to extremes. Cabbage offers your liver with the side effect some assistance with being lower cholesterol, so there is more than one motivation to incorporate this cruciferous vegetable.

Notwithstanding purifying your liver cabbage will likewise help in offering you some assistance with going to the restroom, which thusly offers you some assistance with expelling the toxics, getting them out of your system so you can begin new.

dandelions

Dandelions

Glad liver, solid life is the adage here, and dandelion root can help you on your journey to a sound liver that does its day by day obligations. This plant is viewed as a weed by most grass lovers, yet it has a few mending properties for the liver, and along these lines ought not be ignored when it comes time for detox.

Dandelion has been utilized to treat liver issues going back many years, yet you don't need to hold up until your liver is in critical straights to get the advantages. Fortifying an effectively solid liver will even now yield a lot of good results and makes it worth investigating dandelion on your mission for a wash down.

garlic

Garlic

Numerous detox diets list garlic as a pivotal bit of the riddle. The reason is that garlic supports up the safe system and in addition assisting the liver. One fortunate thing about garlic is that you can up your admission of it without worrying if your body is going to get accustomed to it or develop a resistance.

One other positive angle is that it can add flavor to generally flat nourishments that you'll be eating on your detox program. In any case, in the event that you don't care for the essence of garlic you can at present get its advantages since it comes in supplement structure.

ginger

Ginger

This is one root whose restorative worth goes back to old Chinese civic establishments, and one that is still accepted to offer numerous medical advantages. Regularly utilized as a part of a tea or other beverage, you can add it to the dinners you make too. It is thought to help the liver capacity, and has some astringent properties.

Some detox diets request that you bite on ginger root. You might likewise find that adding it to boiling hot water improves the water taste. Fundamentally any way you can consider it get it into your system will be advantageous, particularly in case you're experiencing a greasy liver brought about by an excessive amount of liquor, or an excess of lethal sustenances and beverages.

grapefruit

Grapefruit

The fiber and the supplement rich juices in a grapefruit pack a decent detox punch and can truly get your body vigorously to the extent detoxing goes. It's about flooding the body with great things for it while offering it some assistance with dislodging the terrible things. The impacts of grapefruit on weight reduction are settled, and one reason might be a result of the way it makes the liver consume fat.

The huge takeaway on grapefruit is that it gets your liver started up and good to go, while implanting whatever is left of your organs with supplement loaded natural product juice. It's a victor with regards to detox nourishments.

green tea

Green Tea

Green tea is regularly considered as an extraordinary expansion to any detox program due to its high cancer prevention agent esteem. Cancer prevention agents are useful in light of the fact that they will search out and murder free radicals before they can do any harm. This is an extraordinary refreshment to drink once a day for this component alone.

Getting into a sound perspective is a matter of feeling like you're doing what's best for your body. It can be something as straightforward as substituting green tea for colas, juices, and different teas with the goal that you can really be profiting your body from a refreshment as opposed to harming it.

kale

Kale

Dr. Oz incorporates kale in his 48 Hour Weekend Cleanse and suggests mixing it up in a shake. In any case you get it into your body, the advantages are that it contains a lot of supplements, furthermore goes about as an approach to flush out the kidneys, an arrangement of organs that should be rinsed on any great detox exertion.

This vegetable is so bravo that it is frequently prescribed to patients that are taking after a specialist suggested diet when battling kidney sickness. It's stuffed with such a large number of cancer prevention agents and has calming properties also, also the greater part of the vitamins and minerals it contains.

lemongrass

Lemongrass

This is a herb that is utilized as a part of Thailand and different parts of the world as a characteristic approach to wash down a few organs on the double. It helps the liver as well as the kidneys, the bladder, and the whole digestive tract. Advantages of utilizing it as a part of your cooking, or drinking it as a tea incorporate a superior appearance, better dissemination, and better absorption.

It is frequently utilized as a tea as a part of the universe of detoxing, and there are a few formulas you can attempt until you discover one that suits your tastes best.

lemons

Lemons

Lemons and lemon juice are regularly said while detoxing, and there's even a couple Lemon Detox Diets gliding around out there. It's just an issue of adding lemon juice to water and drinking it. It should flush toxics from your body. A few individuals include cayanne pepper and sweeten it with sugar, however sugar is not prescribed in case you're attempting to get a detoxifying impact from it.

It assists with your assimilation and you can drink some boiling point water with lemon included request to set up your digestive system for that day's worth of effort.

olive oil

Olive Oil

Some liver purges out there call for olive oil blended with natural product juice so as to trigger your liver to cancel its gallstones. In any case, beside that olive oil ought to be your go-to oil for use in cooking when you're attempting to detox the body. That is on the grounds that it has a ton of solid properties, and settles on for a superior decision of fat than a large portion of your different alternatives.

Simply make sure not to cook with it at high warmth. Use it as a serving of mixed greens dress to offer things such as dull verdant greens some assistance with going down.

ocean growth

Ocean growth

This most likely doesn't enter your menu unless it's wrapped around a bit of sushi, yet ocean growth has a huge amount of supplements and cancer prevention agents in it. In case you're attempting to get more detox sustenances into the body, don't go for the nori they used to hold together a sushi move, you'll need to run with kelp rather to receive the most in return and maintain a strategic distance from the salt that is added to the dried nori.

The kelp is utilized as a part of Asian food and can regularly be found in soups.

Chapter 9

Drug detoxification

The medication detoxification and withdrawal procedures are vital initial phases in characterizing an individual's medication treatment arrangement. Regularly the impacts of medications on the cerebrum excuse proceeded with use and skew generally decision making ability, so having a time of no medication use is essential in understanding that individual to a steady perspective.

The Substance Abuse and Mental Health Services Administration's (SAMHSA) TIP 45 on medication detox takes note of that this period is a "window of chance" for a person in both individual and medicinal emergencies to consider further treatment. Amid detox, a someone who is addicted can clear his or her head and consider tentative arrangements for treatment. The thought is to get the person to start to perceive the habit and diminish and take out medication use.

What Is Detox?

Detox is a progression of intercessions that are intended to oversee withdrawal side effects and intense inebriation, as characterized by SAMHSA. Detox is partitioned from substance misuse treatment; it is a forerunner for it. Now and again it can keep going for a couple of days, yet for others, detox might continue for a couple of months.

Fates of Palm Beach has detoxification pros who can help you effectively treat withdrawal indications and get you into a treatment plan that is separately planned because of you. Since detox does not comprehend the passionate, social, mental, and intellectual issues connected with dependence, it is exceptionally suggested that you seek after a long haul treatment arrangement.

Ventures of Drug Detox

There are three stages to detoxification that, before the end, ought to in a perfect world move the person into an inpatient or outpatient recuperation arrangement.

1. Assessment

All together for a fitting treatment plan to be powerful, it is basic to precisely analyze and evaluate a man's fixation. The assessment stage accomplishes more than distinguish the habit and the level of utilization; it is additionally useful in deciding any hidden therapeutic or mental conditions or inconveniences that might be co-happening alongside the medication misuse.

2. Adjustment

Adjustment is the procedure by which a man starts withdrawal from medications. The objective personality a primary concern for this stage is to acquire a medication free state. Pharmaceuticals can be endorsed amid this stage to help with the compulsion process, particularly if the client has a background marked by overwhelming use. Once the individual has accomplished a condition of parity, in a manner of speaking, and contemplations balance out, a genuine acknowledgment and affirmation of fixation can start. This opens the ways to recuperation treatment and the client's part simultaneously.

3. Encouraging Entry Into Drug Treatment

It is accounted for that an extensive number of people experiencing detox don't look for further treatment for substance misuse habit. While thinking for this shifts from individual to individual, one thing is sure: Those who complete medication free treatment regularly have higher achievement rates for substance restraint. There is an accentuation on habit instruction and duty to temperance. Once this stage is finished, a man can proceed with an office's medication treatment arrangement in either an inpatient or outpatient setting.

It is not very late to look for treatment for your compulsion. In the event that dependence is controlling your life or the life of somebody you know, call Futures of Palm Beach today. We have a particular enslavement treatment office and qualified experts devoted to your prosperity. You can converse with a qualified clinician who can best figure out what alternatives are accessible to you and how you can push ahead with accomplishing a medication free life.

Chapter 10

Cancer and detox

On chemicals and malignancy, a German prominent oncologist says that tumor is created by natural toxics. Others concur. While there are clearly different issues, organisms, infections, hereditary qualities, and so forth., the most critical on the planet that could have prompted the blast of disease in the most recent 100 years change has been the presentation of a huge number of items chemicals in nature. Chemicals that have never been presented to. That our bodies don't know how to handle. The connection between dangerous chemicals and malignancy gets to be clearer the more we are encompassed by them.

Colman your body's resistances and growth creates. Lamentably, if industry and government control have their direction, they might even turn out to be more regrettable.

Biotechnology organizations have been forcefully advancing the utilization of hereditarily altered sustenances. It is a budgetary gold mine for them. Sadly, there are a few issues with GM nourishments. Indeed, even researchers at the FDA opposed until the political weight from the top endorsed. Each autonomous study has demonstrated issues with eating hereditarily adjusted sustenances. the irregular development of cells being high on the rundown. What's more, no big surprise.

Jeffrey Smith, writer of Seeds of Deception SeedsOfDeception.com composes:

"The worry is that the" promoter "is utilized as a part of hereditarily changed nourishments could get exchanged to microscopic organisms or inside organs. The promoters demonstration like a light switches, for all time turning on qualities that may somehow or another be killed. Researchers they trust this could make unusual wellbeing impacts, including development of conceivably pre-destructive cells found in creature bolstering concentrates on specified previously.

"Milk from rBGH-treated cows contains an expanded measure of the hormone IGF-1, which is one of the most elevated danger variables connected with bosom tumor and prostate growth, among others. Soy sensitivities soar in half in the UK, agreeing with the presentation of GM soya imports from the US "

Sustenances are not required to be marked as GM foods.The best way to ensure you are not eating nourishments that have been hereditarily altered is eating natural sustenances or named non-GMO sustenances. Eating natural nourishment will likewise decrease the measure of chemicals that are eating.

Kinds of toxics in your body

There are a few kinds of dangerous gatherings in the body that should be tended to when managing disease chemicals and connection to battle tumor. To start with is the deviation brought about by toxics in the cells because of abundance acridity in the blood, and the failure to discharge toxics into the cells therefore cell lethality.

The accompanying is the overwhelming metal and substance harmfulness that originates from years of introduction to exceptionally lethal substantial metals and chemicals. While numerous originate from nature, silver amalgam fillings, numerous antibodies and different medications put mercury and different toxics in our body. Most huge fish have elevated amounts of mercury. Abnormal amounts of overwhelming metals change the insusceptible system, and ought to be dealt with when battling malignancy.

And after that there is the dangerous development in the colon of undigested nourishments and solidified fecal matter. Supplement retention is interfered, and toxics sitting in that wreckage rotting are reabsorbed by the body. This makes a consistent strain on the invulnerable system, and an extra weight on the detoxification systems of the body. colon purifying needs to happen making a course for good wellbeing.

The chlorinated water and the Cancer

Pathogens in water have prompted numerous maladies. In any case, did you realize that place him in the water to refine it might be the reason for their growth (and coronary illness)?

The French, with their low rates of growth devour OPC and resveratrol in red wine, red wine is renowned for its medical advantages. There is another side of their lower rates of growth that the vast majority don't know ...

The French don't drink chlorinated water. They Ozonate their water to clean it.

Does this have any kind of effect? Completely.

"We are persuaded ... that there is a relationship in the middle of disease and chlorinated water."

Therapeutic College of Wisconsin examination group

We don't utilize substance chlorine since it is sheltered, we utilize it since it is modest. Basically still place chlorine in the water before drinking. The long haul impacts of chlorinated drinking water are an illustration of the awful chemicals and tumor join.

By US Council ecological quality, "Tumor hazard among individuals drinking chlorinated water is 93% higher than among those whose water does not contain chlorine."

It can bring about coronary illness part as well. Dr. Joseph Price composed an exceptionally disputable book in the sixties entitled Coronaries/Cholesterol/Chlorine, and presumed that nothing can discredit the indisputable actuality that the essential reason for atherosclerosis, heart assaults and stroke it is chlorine.

Dr. Cost later headed a study with chickens as guineas pig, where two gatherings of a few hundred feathered creatures were seen amid their whole development. Join chemicals and malignancy was going to be tried ...

One gathering was given water with chlorine and the other without. The gathering raised with chlorine, when autopsied, demonstrated some level of heart or circulatory ailment in each example, the gathering without had no occurrence of the malady. The gathering without chlorine became quicker, bigger and showed fiery wellbeing.

This study was generally welcomed in the poultry business, is still utilized as a source of perspective today. Thus, most expansive poultry makers use dechlorinated water.

At the point when chlorine is added to our water, consolidated with other common mixes to shape trihalomethanes (chlorination repercussions), or THMs. These chlorine repercussions trigger the creation of free radicals in the body, bringing on cell harm, and are profoundly cancer-causing.

"In spite of the fact that centralizations of these cancer-causing agents (THMs) are low, it is unequivocally these low levels that tumor researchers accept are in charge of the larger part of human malignancies in the United States." The Environmental Defense Fund

Dr. Robert Carlson, a regarded analyst at the University of Minnesota, aggregates it up by saying, "Chlorine is the best crippler and killer of cutting edge times!"

Bosom malignancy, which now influences one in eight ladies in North America, has as of late been connected with the gathering of chlorine mixes in the bosom tissue. A study did in Hartford Connecticut, the first of its kind in North America, found that:

"Ladies with bosom tumor have a half to 60% larger amounts of organochlorines (chlorination side effects) in their bosom tissue than ladies without bosom disease."

Not just chlorinated drinking water that is the issue.

Up to 66% of our presentation to chlorine it is because of inward breath of steam and skin ingestion while showering. A warm shower opens the pores of the skin and permits the quick retention of chlorine and different chemicals in the water.

The steam breathe in while showering can contain up to 50 times the level of synthetic than faucet water because of the way that the majority of chlorine and different contaminants are vaporized speedier and at a lower temperature than water substances. Inward breath is a medium a great deal more hurtful type of introduction since chlorine gas (chloroform) we breathe in goes straightforwardly into the circulation system.

"Showering is associated as the essential driver with raised levels of chloroform in about each home due to chlorine in the water."

Dr. Spear Wallace, USA Environmental Protection Agency.

On the off chance that you wash up utilizing chlorinated water and growth is, introducing a shower channel plainly to expel chlorine from your shower water it bodes well.

Different wellsprings of poison

During the time spent disposing of lethal presentation however much as could be expected on account of the chemicals and tumor join, it is important to restrain introduction to chemicals on your floor coverings and dividers of your home. Unless as of now put extraordinary push to have a house free of chemicals, formaldehyde and numerous different chemicals have been outgassing dangerous exhaust in yours for quite a long time. Hulda Clark, in his books on the battle against malignancy and different ailments, suggests that every single halted cover, boards and dividers taken out and supplanted, et cetera - on the off chance that you need to beat growth. really radical things. A less overpowering arrangement would be to acquire a photocatalyst air channel. Utilizing innovation created by NASA, which puts out atoms interfacing with unstable natural mixes, chemicals put out via rugs, and so on and changes in carbon particles and safe water.

individual consideration things, for example, cleanser, conditioner and skin moisturizer frequently contain fixings that build the over-burden of chemicals your invulnerable system ought to dispose of it. Take a stab at utilizing individual consideration things as immaculate and regular, with just synthetic recorded in the fixings as could be expected under the circumstances to diminish this overhead. The less overpowered their safe system is, the better it can battle growth.

The amassing of toxics in your body lessens cell oxygenation and toxics can harm DNA, bringing on cell change. The key is to ensure cells by ensuring you are taking a lot of cancer prevention agents, quit drinking chlorinated water or scrub down in it, and dispose of the amassing of toxics in your body utilizing sheltered and regular detox.

There are three kinds of detox done, cell detoxification, intestinal detoxification and detox the more extensive body in which we will incorporate detoxification of substantial metals. There is some hybrid here, any detoxifying capacity in more than restricted. What's more, recollect that, it is vital to alkalize the body as that should happen before a considerable measure of detoxification should be possible.

Chapter 11

Alcohol detoxification

On the off chance that a man frequently and vigorously utilizes liquor, he or she has a solid danger of adding to a liquor habit or reliance. At the point when the dependent individual chooses to quit drinking or can't drink for any reason, he or she will probably start encountering detox, regularly described by withdrawal indications that are both physical and mental in nature. These indications can extend from exceptionally gentle to extremely serious.

More often than not, liquor detox will go back and forth with no significant inconveniences, yet in a little number of cases, medicinal issues can happen and prompt ailment or passing. To evade the danger of an "untidy" detox, drunkards who wish to quit drinking are urged to experience the procedure in a controlled, restoratively regulated environment.

Picking an administered restorative detox will help you to guarantee that your cherished one adheres to the detox without backslide as well as keeps away from conceivably dangerous wellbeing issues along the way.

At the point when Does Detoxification Start?

On the off chance that your companion or relative has as of late quit drinking, either deliberately or accidentally, you might be thinking about to what extent it will take before the detoxification process begins. While each individual is distinctive, most people will start encountering withdrawal side effects anywhere in the range of five to 10 hours after they quit drinking. A few individuals don't encounter side effects for quite a long time. Indications are generally the most extreme between days two and three, however they can keep on happening for a few weeks in the wake of drinking discontinuance.

Is Help Needed?

There is no real way to tell for certain how extreme or how mellow a man's involvement with liquor detoxification will be. There are, in any case, a few elements that frequently show the withdrawal will be pretty much serious. In the event that your adored one meets a few of the beneath criteria, serious withdrawal side effects are likely – all the more motivation to get ready for a directed, controlled detox experience:

Devouring a lot of liquor before withdrawal

Great nervousness or the vicinity of another mental issue

Having encountered seizures, incoherence, or different genuine withdrawal manifestations before

Utilization of psychoactive medications

Poor general wellbeing

Points of Interest

poly tranquilize use

Poly-Drug Use: The Effects of Drug Cocktails

First-Time-At-A-12-Step-Meeting

What It's Like to Attend Your First 12-Step Meeting

bill to require plug calm living area

Picking a Recovery Residence: Benefits of Sober Living

How Is Alcohol Detox?

Liquor detoxification is diverse for every individual regarding the particular side effects experienced, when they start, to what extent they last, and how they extreme they are in the meantime. When all is said in done, be that as it may, generally experienced liquor withdrawal manifestations might include:

Feeling discouraged and/or on edge

Compelling tiredness

Serious liquor desires

Sentiments of anxiety

A powerlessness to rest

Bountiful sweating

Muscle and general body shortcoming

Body shaking (can influence part or the majority of the body)

Facial tremors

Sentiments of frenzy and blame

Queasiness

At the point when a man is detoxing in a sheltered, medicinal environment, he or she is typically seen all day and all night and offered drugs to simplicity withdrawal manifestations and agony. At the point when not in a therapeutic setting, the best thing you can do is be watchful for any strange manifestations and attempt to make your adored one as agreeable as would be prudent.

Serious side effects of liquor withdrawal that might show a requirement for medicinal consideration include:

Being excessively energized or fomented

Seizures

Mental perplexity

Running a fever

Chapter 12

Exercise for detoxification

Activity is essential for staying solid. It keeps muscles solid, smolders calories, looks after adaptability, increments oxygen consuming limit and offers a pleasurable endorphin discharge. An additional advantage, and one not regularly talked about, is that practice really helps your body to detoxify itself.

What is Detoxification?

Detoxification is the purging of the interior organs of the body from ecological contaminations, sustenance waste, harms, destructive microbes and different substances, for example, liquor, solutions and parasites. The human body is intended to dispose of waste. The organs of detoxification incorporate the colon, liver, lungs, kidneys, skin and lymph organs.

How Detoxification occurs

Your body is continually detoxifying itself.The most evident path is through killing waste by means of urinating or having a defecation. This is restricted your digestive system disposes of unneeded dangerous waste. This happens routinely for just about everybody, and the purging is finished by the colon and kidneys.

The lungs sift through toxics and garbage noticeable all around we inhale before the oxygen is consumed by the blood and taken to the muscles of the body. The skin is our biggest organ. Waste is dispensed with by the skin through sweating. Frequently when the other detoxifying organs are bargained, toxics will start to get through the skin, appearing as skin inflammation, rashes, imperfections, pimples or bruises. The liver is a perplexing organ that helps the body to either utilize or dispose of metabolic waste and natural toxics and substances.

Lymph is an unmistakable liquid that courses through the body containing white platelets. The lymph system is comprised of hubs, which go about as channels, and vessels. The lymph gathers undesirable "trash" in the body, for example, fats, microbes and other destructive materials and channels them through the lymph hubs. The lymph system is like the circulatory system with the exception of there is no "pump" to offer the lymph some assistance with circulating through the body. The lymph system depends entirely on the body's developments for flow.

Why Exercise is Good For Detoxification

Activity is an essential part of any detoxification program. Moving the body makes the conditions for the body to inhale, extend, flow and sweat. It is a smart thought to drink bunches of water amid a detox period, so the skin can sweat and the kidneys can adequately channel toxics. By expanding your water admission, and in addition expanding your heart and breathing rate, your body can all the more successfully flush out undesirable toxics, fats and waste.

How Exercise Detoxifies the Body

Exercise helps the body's organs of disposal to work ideally basically by making them go. Moving the body courses both blood and lymph. The more they flow, the more the liver and lymph hubs can carry out the employment of purging and filtering the blood and lymph.

The digestive system functions admirably and all the more frequently with steady work out. When you practice you inhale profoundly with your lungs. The oxygen that you take in voyages however the blood to the cerebrum and muscles. The lungs expand their ability as the heart muscle becomes more grounded, and they deliver and emit carbon dioxide as a waste result of high-impact exercise. The skin is washed down from the back to front by the purging procedure of sweat. Numerous toxics can be disposed of through the skin by sweating.

Another way practice detoxifies the body is by decreasing the body's subcutaneous greasy tissue. Toxics get put away in the greasy tissue of the body. Along these lines, when greasy tissue is diminished as an aftereffect of vigorous activity, the toxics are discharged and can be disposed of through the purifying organs.

Kinds of Exercise for Detox

Tender, low-force vigorous activity is useful for detox since it gets the body moving, heart pumping and the lungs breathing profoundly however inside of the fat-smoldering zone. Running, strolling, bicycling, moving and swimming are cases of high-impact exercise. Attempt to practice at a pace at which you can inhale equitably and carry on a discussion. Yoga stances are likewise helpful in light of the fact that some are particular for detoxifying certain organs. A few kinds of yoga, Pilates and hand to hand fighting include a vigorous part too.

Bouncing back (skipping on a smaller than normal trampoline) is particularly useful for practicing amid detox in light of the fact that the low-affect movement takes into account astounding incitement of the lymph system. For best results pick a type of activity that you appreciate and begin gradually. Exercise for no less than 20 minutes a few times each week.

Chapter 13

Natural herbs for detoxification
ght you want to feel like a million bucks?

I for one trust that getting to be solid is a procedure which incorporates diet, exercise, great rest and successful anxiety administration. Be that as it may, it is impractical to dependably do all that you have to do to be sound.

Tragically, we likewise live in a period where the toxics in our surroundings can overpower our bodies. Natural toxics, plastics, the contamination created by a lot of carbon noticeable all around, metals, and all the nourishment toxics from pesticides, added substances and colors add to lethal anxiety in our bodies and welcome sickness.

If not managed, toxics will bring about infections that will be ceaseless and likely costly. One arrangement is to detox routinely: in the spring and fall. Another is to take detox herbs all the time. I have gathered a rundown of great herbs that I have utilized for over 10 years that are amazing for lessening toxics in the body and keeping up parity and wellbeing.

Keeping in mind the end goal to frequently detox you have to comprehend what you have to do and what will take care of business.

Mangistha.

To have a solid safe system, you have to clean the lymphatic system, which is the seat of our safe system. The lymphatic system is everywhere on our bodies. It begins in our intestinal divider. It is likewise found in the skin and the majority of our organs where it goes about as a poisonous waste evacuation system. There is a solid relationship between our processing and our invulnerable systems which implies that when the lymphatic system is traded off, our resistant systems can't carry out their occupations. The herb most appropriate for supporting our lymphatic system is manjistha.

Turmeric.

The strength of our digestive system influences our safe system. The bodily fluid film of the gut, a part of the lymph system is traded off by digestive irregular characteristics. These uneven characters which can be brought about by toxics, diet decisions, anxiety and way of life show either as stoppage or loose bowels relying upon whether the lopsided characteristics are drying or making clog. Regular components can add to the irregular characteristics. These lopsided characteristics meddle with our safe working. Turmeric is a herb that assists with this.

Beets

and fenugreek thin the bile. At the point when there is clog in the bodily fluid films of the digestive tract, toxics don't get prepared by the guts. Rather they go down to the liver which thickens the bile which thusly makes clog in the bile and pancreatic channels. The outcome is that fats can't be processed, fat solvent toxics can't be handled and digestive compounds are not as accessible to carry out their occupation. This bargains both the resistant system and absorption. Beets and fenugreek bolster the body's bile as characteristic supplements or as a major aspect of a supper.

Guduchi

rinses the liver with the goal that it can prepare fat solvent toxics so they don't wind up put away in fat cells all through the body.

Shilajit

is known for helping cell recovery. When you have a development of lethality in the body, your cells will be malnourished. Cell recovery restores sustenance and vitality to the cells of the body. Shilajit is the herb for reviving the cells.

Gymnema sylvestre equalizations the glucose which counteracts diabetes. Regardless of the possibility that you devour little sugar, it is in such a large number of sustenances, that you might in any case have a glucose irregularity. Glucose levels when balanced out make it less demanding it use fat stores as fuel for the body, notwithstanding keeping a long haul interminable sicknesses. Gymnena is a brilliant herb for balancing out glucose.

Ginger is an incredible herb for restoring absorption. At the point when toxics hinder the procedure of processing and when the digestive proteins have been debilitated, they require help to restore their working. Ginger will empower the digestive system.

Triphala is one of the most established home grown definitions. It incorporates amalaki, bibhitaki, and haritaki, three detox herbs that backing all systems of the body. Triphala can be utilized as a mellow purgative and it is protected to be utilized consistently as a tender balancer to the body.

Neem is a marvel herb from the neem tree. It is most generally known as a herb for the skin and dental wellbeing. In any case, it is additionally antibacterial, antifungical, against viral, germ-free, hostile to diabetic, and blood cleaning, and has numerous other functional employments.

None of these detox herbs are costly and all can offer you some assistance with removing so as to improve your personal satisfaction toxics from you body and feeling like a million bucks.

Maria Hill is the website admin for HSP Health and HSP Health Blog. She is quite a while meditator, reiki expert, understudy of option wellbeing and Ayurveda. Maria is a unique painter at Infinite Shape furthermore extremely intrigued by creature and human rights and the earth. Interface with her on Facebook, Twitter, Google+ or the HSP Health Google+ page.

Compose For Us!

Supported Links

12 Unexpected Benefits of Drinking Hot Water

Wellbeing Lifestyleby Tegan Jones

I imagine that the majority of us know at this point water is vital to our survival. We've presumably likewise all heard specialists say that drinking approximately eight glasses a day is perfect. In any case, what the vast majority don't know is that warm water and boiling hot water have some restrictive advantages of their own that you can't get when you drink water chilly. Here are 12 advantages of drinking boiling point water:

1. Weight reduction

High temp water is incredible for keeping up a sound digestion system, which is the thing that you need in case you're attempting to shed a couple of kilos. The most ideal approach to do this is to kick begin your digestion system at a young hour in the morning with a glass of high temp water and lemon. To really sweeten the deal, boiling point water will separate the fat tissue (otherwise known as muscle to fat quotients) in your body.

2. Helps with Nasal and Throat Congestion

Drinking heated water is a fantastic regular solution for colds, hacks and a sore throat. It breaks down mucus furthermore expels it from your respiratory tract. All things considered, it can give alleviation from a sore throat. It additionally helps in clearing nasal blockage.

3. Menstrual Cramps

High temp water can likewise help in lessening menstrual issues. The warmth of the water has a quieting and mitigating impact on the muscular strength, which in the long run can cure issues and fits.

4. Body Detoxification

High temp water is fabulous for helping your body to detox. When you drink boiling hot water, your body temperature starts to rise, which brings about sweat. You need this to happen in light of the fact that it discharges toxics from your body and wash down it legitimately. For ideal results, include a press of lemon before drinking.

5. Avoids Premature Aging

There's a reason you ought to need to clear your group of toxics: they make you age quicker. Additionally, drinking heated water repairs the skin cells that build the flexibility of your skin and are influenced by hurtful free radicals. In this way, your harmed skin gets to be smoother.

6. Averts Acne and Pimples

The advantages for your skin simply continue coming. High temp water profound purifies your body and wipes out the main drivers of skin break out related contaminations.

7. Hair Health and Vitality

Drinking boiling point water is additionally useful for acquiring delicate, glossy hair. It stimulates the nerve endings in your hair roots and makes them dynamic. This is helpful for getting back the characteristic essentialness of your hair and keeping it solid.

8. Advances Hair Growth

Initiating the bases of your hair has another included advantage—development! The boiling point water advances the customary movement of the roots and thusly quickens the development of your hair.

9. Averts Dandruff

Chapter 14

Natural ways of detoxification

Purging weight control plans, herbs, and fasting projects might appear like an advanced wellbeing drift however social orders have utilized common purifying strategies to detoxify the body for many years. Numerous religions really urge individuals to quick as a method for purifying both the body and the psyche for otherworldly practices. Poisonous and contaminated sustenance systems, air and water, and environment make purging the colon, liver and different organs more imperative now than any time in recent memory. The weight of over-contamination might be in charge of pernicious impacts on the safe system, a situation which makes us very vulnerable to unending degenerative illnesses, for example, a few types of growth, coronary illness, diabetes, Alzheimer's ailment and the sky is the limit from there.

This article will separate a few of the present strategies and sustenances that help the body, actually, accomplish a detoxified state. Try to dependably keep away from refined nourishments, sugars, MSG, yeast, dairy items, caffeine and chocolate, soy, peanuts, liquor and non-entire grain starches while doing any kinds of rinse or quick.

Common Detox Methods

Liver wash down Regimes for purifying the liver ought to fuse all the more intense greens and chlorophyll squeezes, for example, wheat-grass and dandelion greens. Other liver-upbeat sustenances incorporate carrots, celery, limes, lemons and beets. Flavors that offer purifying consequences for the liver incorporate turmeric, rosemary, cayenne, cumin and curry. Maintain a strategic distance from espresso, milk and soft drinks, rather settle on decontaminated water and/or squeezed apple. To bolster your purifying endeavors, add Livatrex to a gallon of squeezed apple or water and take after these liver purging guidelines.

Oxygen colon purge One of the best regular detox strategies is a six or seven day wash down utilizing refined water, natural/crude apple juice vinegar, aloe vera juice, Oxy-Powder and a probiotic supplement. This wash down is a brisk and viable approach to clean your digestive tract. Here are my suggested guidelines for doing a colon purify.

Candida wash down This is intended to expel candida from the body by uprooting all nourishments containing yeast or aged sustenances. This eating regimen requires keeping away from all types of sugar (counting leafy foods squeeze), every refined flour and wheat items, any nourishments containing yeast, and in addition every characteristic sweetener, for example, agave nectar or crude nectar. Amid a candida purge you ought to likewise keep away from mixed beverages, dried natural products, mushrooms, cheddar, salted vegetables and soy sauce. Natural oregano oil and Latero-Flora are additionally to a great degree viable against candida.

Destructive living being scrub There are numerous herbs you can take to slaughter off undesirable intestinal infestations that might be influencing your wellbeing. Wormwood, dark walnut body, clove and American wormseed are four herbs that make a threatening domain inside your intestinal tract for attacking living beings, and murder living beings that might as of now arrive. Taking a probiotic supplement will likewise flush out any unwelcome guests. Here is my prescribed purifying directions for unsafe creatures.

Fluid purify An amazing approach to scrub the body while as yet keeping up vitality levels. A fluid purge includes the utilization of crisp natural foods grown from the ground juices, pureed soups, miso soup, smoothies, oils, for example, flax, hemp, coconut, sesame or pumpkin seed oil, and new, clean water.

Harmful metal wash down Most individuals have elevated amounts of lethal metals, for example, mercury, aluminum, cadmium and lead in their body. It is prescribed that people perform two washes down every year to flush these toxics out of the body to dodge long haul aggregation. Find out around a simple at home strategy for purifying dangerous metals from the body here.

Crude/antacid sustenances purge This is an impermanent rinse utilizing uncooked foods grown from the ground, consolidated with littler measures of crude nuts, seeds and sprouts. This is a superb approach to detoxify the colon, liver and other real systems. It lessens the body's have to continually endeavor to alkalize the acidic way of the blood, from eating a present day, non-soluble eating regimen. Take in more about the advantages of a crude nourishment diet.

Juice fasts-This comprises of expending just naturally squeezed foods grown from the ground for one to three days or more. Accommodating, purging foods grown from the ground incorporate apples, carrots, beets, ginger root, spinach, pears, celery, kale, cabbage, pineapple, cranberry, and other dull verdant greens. Citrus natural products are typically maintained a strategic distance from while fasting. Natural products of the soil are best, and also newly squeezed foods grown from the ground (not packaged).

Kitcheree purge A kitcheree wash down is an antiquated Ayurvedic strategy for purifying the body through what is known as a "mono-diet." In a kitcheree scrub, you can eat a super-basic eating regimen of mung beans, cooked vegetables, basmati rice and flavors. This eating routine offers an interim alleviation to the digestive system, and adds to general detoxification, particularly when consolidated with purging herbs.

Clove for purging

Purging flavors Coupling a sound natural eating regimen with the utilization of purifying flavors is a mellow method for making change in the body. Purging flavors to add to your eating routine incorporate cinnamon, oregano, turmeric, cumin, cilantro, fenugreek, ginger, fennel, cayenne pepper, dark pepper, clove, parsley and rosemary.

Expert wash down This detox strategy comprises of an eating routine made just out of crisply crushed lemon juice, natural evaluation B maple syrup, cayenne pepper and spring water. While this can be a viable strategy for both liver and colon purifying, I would even now prescribe doing an oxygen colon purge and a liver/gallbladder wash down in the meantime.

Which of these have you attempted and what were your encounters? If it's not too much trouble share your criticism!

On the off chance that you would prefer not to do a more amazing kinds of wash down, you've done one and need to move to a more beneficial way of life or your officially pregnant, the accompanying tips won't just offer your body some assistance with ridding itself of toxics, yet will set you up with propensities for a sound way of life.

1. Drink heaps of water

Our body is made of cells. These cells should be hydrated to work legitimately. I went by a naturopath worried about my vitality levels and the principal thing she asked me was, "how much water do you drink?" After advising her my terribly low normal, she exhorted me to drink 1/2 my body weight in ounces each and every day.

Water is imperative for keeping up vitality levels and for flushing out toxics. Amid pregnancy, hydration is vital for keeping up amniotic liquid volume and your own particular blood volume. Without it, your heart is compelled to work harder, expanding your heart rate.

For included purifying, include some lemon juice or lemon key oil (ensure it's protected to expend) in your water. Citrus helps in the disposal of toxics.

2. Sweat

Another approach to free your group of toxics is to sweat it out. Moving your body is awesome for your wellbeing in any case, yet it can likewise offer you some assistance with getting free of developed toxics. Expand exercise that makes you sweat. My most loved approach to sweat out toxics is by doing Bikram (hot) yoga – I've never sweat such a great amount in my life. However, with the abundance sweating, recollect to drink loads of water to flush out toxics.

You can likewise do this by going to your most loved spa. Any reason to go to a spa, isn't that so? Sitting in a steam room or sauna will likewise make them sweat out the terrible stuff. While you're grinding away, plan a back rub.

3. Trench the Junk

This is tremendous. Sustenance is an indispensable part of a solid way of life thus it is essential to eat as " clean" as could reasonably be expected. What does eating clean resemble? Loads of new foods grown from the ground. Ideally natural, however not every one of them must be.

Meat and dairy ought to originate from grass-encouraged, bovines, ideal from a nearby rancher (who you know without a doubt is just bolstering his cows grass). Eggs are a superb wellspring of crucial vitamins, minerals, protein and sound fat. Unfenced chicken eggs can be found in a few stores, yet numerous individuals who raise chickens additionally offer their abundance eggs. Check Craigslist for that.

Sustaining your body with sound fats gives the building pieces to very much adjusted hormones. Margarine (from those stunning grass-bolstered dairy animals) and natural coconut oil are superb and tasty nourishments for ensuring you're getting satisfactory measures of the right kinds of fat.

Discover formulas that will offer you some assistance with incorporating these nourishment into your life and attempt to keep it basic. The purpose of this change is to make propensities forever, which won't happen on the off chance that you have to cook with a huge amount of fixings that are elusive. In case you're searching for more help on eating a sustaining, entire nourishments diet, look at our sister site, Modern Alternative Kitchen.

4. Use Natural Cleaners

We have toxics surrounding us – our homes alone have chemicals in the paint, rug and cleaners. Figuring out how to make your own cleaners is an awesome, straightforward approach to decrease your presentation to hurtful toxics. Numerous formulas require these fixings:

Borax

Preparing pop

Vinegar

Fundamental oils

Lemon juice

Washing pop

Castile cleanser

Utilize these fixings to make your own clothing cleanser, dishwasher cleanser, latrine cleaner, generally useful cleaner and significantly more.

5. Use Herbs

Herbs can be a useful piece of purifying your body. Be that as it may, as with most things in life, it will work better for you in the event that you can keep it straightforward. Luckily, numerous purging herbs are normal ones that you'd find in your kitchen: garlic, ginger root, cayenne pepper and parsely leaf.

Garlic is a characteristic anti-microbial that purifies the blood and helps the invulnerable system.

Cayenne cleans the blood, builds sweating and liquid disposal.

Ginger root fortifies course and sweating.

Parsley leaf is a diuretic that flushes the kidneys. (Keep away from if breastfeeding – it is likewise useful for bringing down your milk supply).

What's more, these can all be effortlessly consolidated into your eating regimen. You can develop your own herbs, or purchase natural herbs here.

Chapter 15

Full body detoxification guide

Detoxification can be a critical technique to bolster the patient amid their recuperating emergency. Similarly as with numerous immune system cases, there are numerous variables. Neurotoxin over-burden is a typical issue that influences numerous patients. The wellspring of neurotoxins might be overwhelming metals, infections, microbes (on account of Lyme), organisms, molds, parasites and protozoans. A portion of the toxics really target, hinder and even harm the sensory system and the detoxification organs. This can assist hinder and obstruct the course for typical discharge, creating a collection of toxics. This outcomes in intracellular harm and further movement of ailment.

In Lyme illness, the microorganisms is a "shrewd" bug which needs to keep up its life inside of the individual. It really conceals itself from the invulnerable system. The Lyme microorganisms is neurotoxic and, with a specific end goal to survive, stops up the lymphatic system and causes the blood to thicken. This prompts poor blood course through the liver and a stickiness to the interstitial liquid. The interstitial liquid is the liquid that showers and feeds the tissue cells. It likewise grabs microorganisms, outside particles, catalysts, proteins, and hormones for handling through the lymphatic system. Notwithstanding the lymphatic system, Lyme likes to go through the collagen more than the blood. Lyme sickness is a systemic disease and it can attack and harm all organs, organs, and systems of our body. Lyme patients are additionally tested by other co-diseases that are regularly disregarded.

In view of its capacity to avoid the resistant system, Lyme makes itself hard to analyze through testing and along these lines hard to outline a compelling treatment convention. Regularly it can cover itself as an alternate malady, for example, Chronic Fatigue Syndrome, Fibromyalgia, Multiple Sclerosis, Parkinson's, Obsessive Compulsive Disorder (OCD), or Amyotrophic Lateral Sclerosis (Lou Gehrig ailment). It is critical for the doctor to determine if Lyme is at a causal level in these maladies. Accepting the patient is being treated with a proper convention, successful detoxification assumes a critical part in taking out the neurotoxins from the body.

At the point when the Lyme is being executed, it creates its own particular neurotoxin in barrier. This in this way stops up the blood, lymph, liver and colon which backs off the detoxification pathways. Furthermore, the length of the patient is in treatment for Lyme, detoxification should be continuous. At the point when the body is overburdened with a harmful burden, the patient may encounter a Herxheimer (Herx) response. One of my patients clarified her Herx responses like an awful aftereffect. She had great weariness, migraines, queasiness, influenza like manifestations, and a shivering sensation all through her body. She likewise saw that her standard side effects were aggravated much. It is amid these scenes, the detoxification process turns out to be much more imperative.

Subsequent to there are various techniques for detoxification, one must choose those which offer the most backing. The two essential pathways of detoxification are: 1) the colon which evacuates strong squanders and 2) the kidneys and bladder which uproots fluid squanders. These pathways have outside end, those being excrement and pee. The liver is likewise an essential detoxification organ for toxics, hormones, and protein and fat digestion system. The pathway for water-solvent toxics is through the pee. Hormones are discharged through bile in the GI tract. The lungs and skin are the optional pathways. The lungs outgas toxics from the circulation system and the skin goes about as a discharge pathway by emitting with pimples, pustules, abscesses or overflowing injuries in the endeavor to expel toxics from the body.

Colon Functions

The elements of the colon (additionally called the internal organ or huge gut) are various. These capacities work extremely well when the intestinal microscopic organisms is of gainful askindsments and in adequate amounts. The colon really makes certain supplements for us, including B 12 and Vitamin K. It retains supplements which may have been missed in the small insides which keeps us supplement thick. Third, it obstructs the ingestion of pathogens and toxics from coming back to the circulatory system. Next, it reabsorbs and reuses water and bile. The water is utilized to keep the body from getting dried out and the bile is reused in assimilation of fats. At last, the colon decays chyme (processed nourishment) into fecal material as the last segment of the life cycle. It is basically our very own manure pit.

Colon Detoxification

For successful end of strong waste, it is critical to have an appropriate tying specialists, for example, fiber or chlorella. This is particularly valid with neurotoxins. One needs to likewise have various every day solid discharges or colon hydrotherapy. Generally the neurotoxins are reabsorbed from the colon once more into the system and redistributed all through the body. This endless loop should be broken.

With any detoxification convention, if the insides are not working productively and viably, this is the primary spot to begin. Likewise, 60 percent of the resistant system is in the digestion systems which is called GALT. This stands for Gut Associated Lymphoid Tissue. Hence a legitimately working gastrointestinal (GI) tract is basic for insusceptible capacity. To keep the entrails working we can utilize colon hydrotherapy, supplements which relax the insides, and, above all, colon reflorastation treatment.

Colon hydrotherapy, likewise called colonics, is the delicate washing out of the digestive organ. Numerous zones have colon specialists, some don't. To locate a skillful specialist, chat with the all encompassing experts in your general vicinity. Colonics are a successful approach to uproot fecal material when there is lethality, stoppage, or poor muscle activity in the colon. It additionally uproots bile which has not been consumed. Amid a colonic, a great part of the fecal material in the 5 feet of internal organs is uprooted. Colonic ought to be directed as required.

At the point when there is lower stomach torment, castor oil packs as per the Edgar Cayce technique are valuable. Utilize a bit of fleece or cotton wool. Immerse it with hexane free castor oil and place the fabric on the stomach area from the base of the ribs to the highest point of the hip bones. It can be secured with a bit of plastic such as a junk sack liner which keeps the oil from ruining our attire or bedding. A warming cushion or heated water jug is set on top of the plastic for the one hour treatment. These are recommended three times each week or as required. More is certainly better and a few patients lay down with the pack covering the stomach area. The wool doesn't should be washed, simply put in a Ziploc® pack until the following application. Extra oil is utilized for every treatment. There are studies which demonstrate that these packs expand the detoxification process, reinforce the invulnerable system and abatement torment. They can be utilized before colonics or as required.

On the off chance that colonics are unrealistic, there are various approaches to expand inside action: magnesium oxide, vitamin C in gem structure, digestive catalysts, or natural supplements, for example, hyssop. These animate the muscle activity of the colon called peristalsis. A periodic utilization of the herbs cascara sagrada or senna is satisfactory in spite of the fact that these are not a favored decision, as they can aggravate the fragile covering of the insides.

At the point when there are unreasonable entrails developments because of looseness of the bowels or fractious gut disorder, it is desirable over start with one colon reflorastation treatment. This treatment is the rectal presentation of probiotics. Because of the acridity of the stomach, most probiotics don't effectively achieve the internal organ. The oral strategy just has a win rate of two to five percent.

However in a rectal application, 100 % of the microscopic organisms are held and thrive in this dull, wet, and warm environment. Along these lines the colon will colonize inside of one hour and balance out in three days. This is called colon reflorastation treatment and can be readministered as regularly as required. This gives fast backing to detoxification.

In my 30 years of private practice, I have consistently tried numerous askindsments of probiotics and have found those which are sheltered, proficient, and viable. This is controlled by a positive reaction on 95% of the considerable number of patients. Along these lines, I have planned an exclusive equation which has twenty askindsments and 50 billion in amount for each application. This gives a fast expansion of microorganisms. For those with compound or natural affectability, every individual microbes can be tried with EAV or Vega testing.

The essentialness of this recipe has demonstrated an essential backing for the GI tract and an optional backing for the liver, kidneys, and invulnerable system. Due to this, the recurrence of colonics can be diminished unless there is incessant blockage or moderate gut travel time.

Entrail travel time is the quantity of hours or days it takes for our nourishment to fly out from our mouth to definite end. We test this with unpopped bits of corn or a substantial serving of beets. When we see the confirmation in the stool, we can decide the measure of time it took to finish the adventure through our digestive tract.

While tending to the recurrence and viability of entrail end, we have to additionally consider parasites. Lyme likes to cover up in parasites. These tiny trespassers may be single adaptable cells, worms, protozoan, contagious spores, or yeasts. While I don't believe that parasites are causal to an infection, I do think they are patrons to the crumbling of the patient's crucial power.

Parasite Detoxification

Most parasites live in the colon where the small digestion tracts interface on the lower right half of the belly. In any case, they can be found in many regions of the body. Numerous specialists release parasites as a sympathy toward those living in underdeveloped countries. In an example of right around 3,000 individuals, 32% tried positive for some kinds of parasitic disease.

Parasites aggravate the coating of the GI tract which obstructs the assimilation of supplements. A characteristic by-result of parasites is corrosive, which can bring about the focal sensory system to wind up languid, harm organs, and separate muscle tissue. In their procedure of development and multiplication, they radiate toxics that influence the liver and kidneys. These detoxification organs then get to be exhausted and lazy. Since parasites impede the development of valuable probiotics, they make a domain that permits yeast to prosper.

An exhaustive parasite detoxification system will address these intruders three ways. In the first place, we utilize a vigorous methodology with a homeopathic cure. Second, a substance strategy is utilized. I favor a tincture of dark walnut. It is best to choose the green structure since it has the most noteworthy centralization of the concoction which influences parasites. Third, there is a mechanical strategy utilizing a sustenance grade type of diatomaceous earth.

Following most parasites have an existence cycle of 21 days, a parasite wash down ought to most recent 23 days or more. A delicate entrail chemical will move the parasites, their trash, and their eggs out all the more rapidly. I lean toward one that is rice based since it is less demanding to dispose of in light of the fact that it stays delicate and elusive.

Liver Functions

When we have a sound colon, it is important to look to the liver. Toxics in the body can open the liver to harm which causes a reduction in liver digestion system. This is called drowsy liver. Manifestations from this kinds of harm incorporate weakness, cerebral pains, obscured vision, expanded fat stockpiling, and hormone unevenness.

Our liver has a focal part in the expulsion of toxics from the body. It additionally detoxifies and discharges hormones into the bile. Another principle capacity of the liver is protein digestion system. At the point when there is diminished blood course through the liver, there can be expanded levels of smelling salts in the blood. One other focal capacity is fat digestion system, especially cholesterol and phospholipids, for example, lecithin. It is accordingly fundamental that our liver stays in ideal working condition.

Liver Detoxification

There is a particular distinction in liver detoxification compounds which exist in the middle of men and ladies. This is because of the stage 1 liver detoxification compound prompted by progesterone. What we should recollect is that it influences our helplessness and result to lethal introduction. Maybe this is a variable which adds to the high frequency rate of a mental imbalance in guys, more than females. Likewise, hereditary changes of the liver detoxification pathways can make our employment considerably more troublesome.

Subsequent to the liver detoxification pathways are perplexing, this article is not about comprehension it. Rather, how about we figure out how to viably bolster this procedure. Squeezing with dark green vegetables, including kale, grain grass, horse feed, and beet greens will bolster progressing every day detoxification. Likewise, search for a nutritious item which has a mix of supplements intended to address both stage 1 and stage 2 detoxification pathways. Start with a little measurement, increment gradually, and shift the dosage as required. We do this to diminish the likelihood of herx and detox responses.

Should this happen or on the off chance that you are feeling dangerous, lazy or slow, consider an espresso douche. They can diminish the heap in the liver. There is a gateway vein which permits the espresso in the rectum and lower colon to quickly enact the liver. It dumps the dangerous burden into the GI tract for evacuation by means of the stool.

A simple strategy for conveyance of espresso is to utilize natural moment espresso in a 4 ounce expendable bowel purge bottle. To begin with, pour off an ounce of the saline arrangement. Include 3 tablespoons of the natural moment espresso to the container. It is then warmed by setting it in some high temp water for a few minutes. Lie on your left side to oversee the purification. Whenever finished, turn onto your back and put a little pad under the bottom. On the off chance that conceivable hold this for five to twenty minutes, longer if conceivable, before ousting the espresso. These might likewise be rehashed as frequently as required. In any case it is essential to occasionally do the colon reflorastation treatment.

Amid espresso purifications we are disturbing the pH (corrosive soluble equalization) of the colon. Our sound microbes are currently attempting to get out the toxics from the liver while having their surroundings not exactly ideal. 24 hours after the espresso bowel purges, oversee another colon reflorastation to further backing our detoxification channels.

Lymphatic System and Function

Since we are keeping the colon and liver in better working request, we have to swing to the lymphatic pathways. This is our insusceptible system. While the skin is the biggest organ of the resistant system, sixty percent of the insusceptible system is in the digestion systems. The lymph vessels are situated close to our corridors and veins. These divert toxics and squanders from the cells. The pathogens are then caught in lymph hubs until they can be annihilated by cells. We can all the more effortlessly feel our lymph hubs in our neck, under our arms, and around the crotch. They likewise encompass our crucial organs, our face and our head.

Lymphatic Detoxification

There are two types of lymphatic seepage treatment: manual and electronically helped. The best and fast strategy is the electronically helped. These medications might last from 30 minutes to a hour and a half. It is essential to not over-burden the system when taking your first treatment. On the off chance that influenza like indications, sickness, or migraines happen, make sure the colon and liver are very much upheld. Longer sessions can be taken when the responses are insignificant or middle of the road.

This type of lymph seepage utilizes far infrared warmth and multi-wave wavering frequencies with honorable gasses. Infrared is a kinds of undetectable light with electromagnetic waves. Research has demonstrated that far infrared beam has a high esteem on human wellbeing. These beams enter into the cells and make a water atom reverberation. It enters the subcutaneous cell layer and raises the temperature. This expansions fine enlargement and dissemination. Right now there is a discharge of blood and congested toxics. This actuates the cells, helps with repair and security of these cells, and advances the development of catalysts.

Notwithstanding the far infrared warmth, we utilize multi-wave wavering frequencies. These depend on quantum material science. At the point when the light vitality is connected to the skin, it builds the stream of both blood and lymphatic liquids. Amid the lymphatic waste treatment, the light is connected to the skin in a methodical example. Toxics are decoupled from the interstitial liquid. They should then go through the lymphatics. In the wake of being handled in the lymph hubs the toxics are discharged in the pee.

This light can likewise be utilized amid colonics as the gut tackles the vitality field and builds the stream of blood and lymph inside of the colon. This expansions detoxification. Whether we do this as a full lymphatic seepage treatment or notwithstanding a colon hydrotherapy, we will have a lessening of toxics and pathogenic material. Normally we will have more beneficial cells.

After a lymphatic waste treatment, it is critical to drink a lot of water and scrub down. One of the most straightforward items to utilize is epsom salt. No less than one pound of epsom salt is added to the shower water. Submerge the body however much as could be expected for 15 to 20 minutes. Utilize a loofah or vegetable brush to altogether brush the skin toward the end of the shower. Other shower items, especially those with EDTA can help with the extra evacuation of toxics and overwhelming metals. Showers might be consolidated into any convention as it fortifies the end of toxics through the skin.

In my private practice, I have come to understand that organization of the colon reflorastation treatment is vital to the lymphatic waste treatment. This should be possible after a colonic or as the lymphatic treatment starts. Along these lines, I have possessed the capacity to totally take out detox responses after the treatment. Something else, patients experience side effects, for example, weakness, influenza like manifestations, cerebral pains, and queasiness.

Detoxification Baths

A detox shower can be as straightforward as the epsom salt shower clarified above or as exhaustive as one utilizing particular hardware. There are a few models accessible which radiate mending frequencies into the water. The unit which I lean toward has four elements. The capable ultrasonic waves offer the body some assistance with recovering from weakness, has a rubbing impact and helps vitality levels as it drives warm profound into the body. This warms the bones and the inside organs while enhancing flow. The mat radiates far infrared beams which make an attractive field to detoxify whatever parts of the body are submerged in the water. It makes ozone from surrounding air and scatters it into the water as air pockets. Thusly, the skin moves the ozone into the circulatory system crippling the toxics. The last component is the negative particles which, similar to a rainstorm, are produced anions to advance cell action and help with the body's capacity to process oxygen.

The advantages of this kind of shower are inside warming, profound purging as it discharges toxics, and the advantages of back rub, for example, inactive activity and unwinding. A run of the mill treatment is 15 minutes and should be possible every so often or up to four times each day.

Other Detoxification Methods

There are various different types of detoxification, including hyperbaric oxygen, ionic foot showers, homeopathic seepage, and intravenous infusions of hydrogen peroxide and supplements. What is basic is to perceive the poisonous issue being experienced.